GENTLE YOGA

ARTHRITIS

Featuring Contributions By

LAURIE SANFORD AND
NANCY FORSTBAUER

D1016246

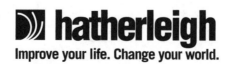

hatherleigh

Improve your life. Change your world.

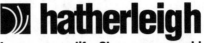

Improve your life. Change your world.

Hatherleigh Press is committed to preserving and protecting the natural resources of the earth. Environmentally responsible and sustainable practices are embraced within the company's mission statement.

Visit us at www.hatherleighpress.com and register online for free offers, discounts, special events, and more.

Gentle Yoga for Arthritis

Library of Congress Cataloging-in-Publication Data is available.
ISBN: 978-1-57826-448-3

DISCLAIMER

Consult your physician before beginning any exercise program. The author and publisher of this book and workout disclaim any liability, personal or professional, resulting from the misapplication of any of the following procedures described in this publication.

Cover Design by Heather Daugherty
Interior Design by Heather Magnan
Photography by Catarina Astrom

Printed in the United States

10 9 8 7 6 5 4 3 2 1

TABLE OF CONTENTS

ACKNOWLEDGMENTS

Hatherleigh Press would like to extend a special thank you to Jo Brielyn—without your hard work and dedication this book would not have been possible.

CHAPTER 1

WHAT IS ARTHRITIS?

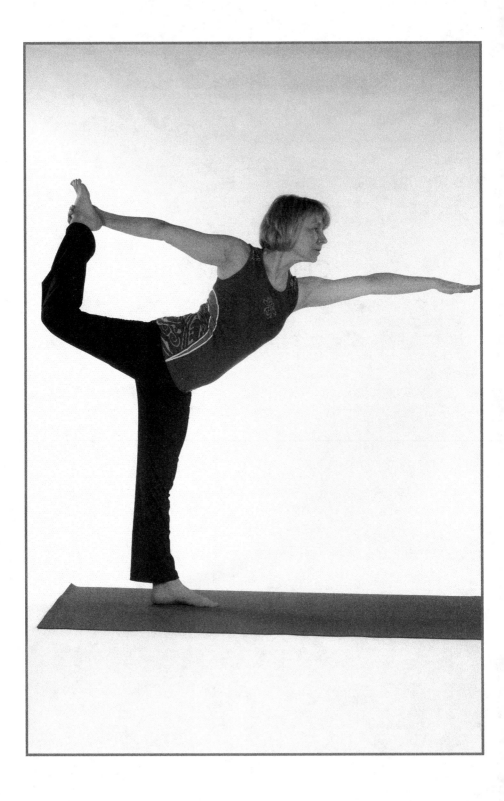

Arthritis is inflammation of the *joints,* which are the locations where bones meet, in one or more areas of the body. The term originates from the Greek word *arthron* meaning "joint" and the Latin word *itis* which means "inflammation". While arthritis is often referred to as one single disease, "arthritis" is actually the term used to encompass more than 100 medical conditions that are identified by inflammation or pain in muscles, joints, or fibrous tissue that surround the joints. These types of conditions are also called *rheumatism* or *rheumatic conditions.* The common denominator among all rheumatic conditions that are considered forms of arthritis is that they all affect the musculoskeletal system, and specifically the joints. Rheumatic conditions are typically characterized by stiffness and pain in or near the joints. Some arthritic conditions (such as lupus and rheumatoid arthritis) may also involve various internal organs and the immune system. Of course, the pattern, location, and severity of the symptoms will be different depending on the form or forms of arthritis affecting the individual.

The Centers for Disease Control and Prevention (CDC) reports that according to a survey conducted in 2013, about 52.5 million adults in the United States had physician-diagnosed arthritis in 2010-2012. That equates to over 1 in every 5 adults in America. Those results showed an increase of 2.5 million from 2007–2009. The new data is consistent with the future projected estimates from the National Health Interview Survey (NHIS) which estimate there will be a staggering 67 million American adults living with arthritis by the year 2030.

What Are the Causes of Arthritis and Who Gets It?

Arthritis is more prevalent among adults, and is often thought of as an aging condition, however people of all ages can be affected by it. Even children are diagnosed with some forms of arthritis.

Since there is such a large group of conditions that are classified as arthritis, the causes and effects are varied. What they all do have in common is the presence of inflammation or pain in muscles, joints, or fibrous tissue that surround the joints.

Here is a more detailed look at five of the most common forms of arthritis: osteoarthritis, rheumatoid arthritis, fibromyalgia, lupus, and gout.

Osteoarthritis

Osteoarthritis affects approximately 27 million adults in the United States and is the most prominent type of arthritis diagnosed in America. *Osteoarthritis* occurs when the *cartilage* (tissue that acts as a cushion at the ends of the bones within the joints) breaks down and erodes.

Then the smooth cartilage surface that would normally act as a shock absorber with the movement of bones around the joints becomes thinner and rougher. In more severe instances of osteoarthritis, all of the cartilage may wear away and cause the bones to constantly grate against each other.

The results of osteoarthritis are pain, inflammation, and sometimes a lack of mobility. Patients with osteoarthritis usually experience a deep aching in and around their joints. They may also feel stiffness in the joints after sitting for a long time or when first getting out of bed. Having swelling in one or more of the joints, or hearing or feeling a crunching of bones rubbing may also happen with osteoarthritis.

The most common areas of the body to be affected by osteoarthritis are the *weight-bearing joints* such as the knees, hips, and ankles. The joints in the feet, hands, and cervical spine are spots where osteoporosis is also likely to occur.

Osteoarthritis generally develops in the joints due to an injury, infection, or simply as a result of the aging process. The risk of developing osteoarthritis may also be greater if you have a family history of the disease.

Rheumatoid Arthritis (RA)

Rheumatoid arthritis (RA) is a progressive inflammatory disease that inflicts damage on the organs and joint tissues. It is caused by a malfunction in the *immune system,* the system in the body that normally protects the body against harmful organisms. When rheumatoid arthritis is present, the immune system instead attacks the membrane lining of the joints. *Rheumatoid arthritis* attacks the synovial membrane and can eventually lead to the destruction of both the bone and cartilage found inside the joints. The *synovial membrane* (also known as *synovium*) is the soft tissue found between the joint capsule and the joint cavity. The result is pain and swelling. It can also lead to deformity and disability if left untreated.

Rheumatoid arthritis differs from osteoarthritis in that it is an autoimmune disease. That means it is a form of arthritis that results from the immune system attacking its own body tissues. Therefore, rheumatoid arthritis can also affect body parts other than joints, like the eyes, mouth, and lungs. Any joint can be affected by RA, but the most common ones are in the wrist and fingers.

Symptoms commonly associated with rheumatoid arthritis are swelling, tenderness, and warmness in joints; stiffness; fatigue; joint pain; fever; and loss of function in the joints.

It is uncertain what causes rheumatoid arthritis to strike in certain individuals. It is believed that genes, environment, and hormones may contribute to the risk of developing this form of arthritis. Rheumatoid arthritis occurs significantly more often in women than men. It also typically strikes when individuals are between the ages of 40 and 60. However, people who are older and even children can also be affected.

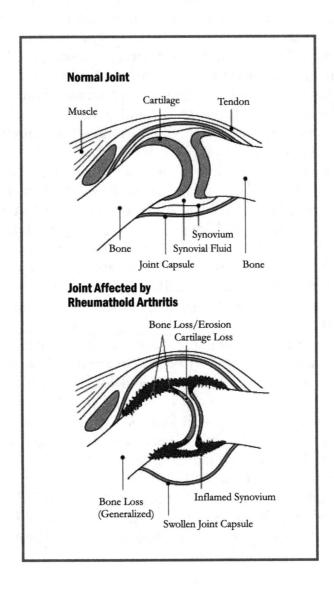

Fibromyalgia

Fibromyalgia (also referred to as *fibromyositis* or *fibrositis*) is a complex *chronic pain disorder* that generally causes long-term fatigue and musculoskeletal pain in joints, tendons, muscles, and other soft tissues throughout the entire body. This sometimes debilitating form of arthritis gets its name from "fibro" which means fibrous tissue (like ligaments and tendons), "my" meaning muscles, and "algia" which means pain.

The National Institute of Arthritis and Musculoskeletal and Skin Diseases (NIAMS) reports that fibromyalgia affects around 5 million people 18 years of age or older in America. Despite the great number of individuals who have fibromyalgia, it is classified as a *syndrome,* not a *disease.* In order to be classified as a disease, there must be a definite cause, or causes, as well as signs and symptoms that are clearly identified. That is not the case with fibromyalgia, which is often called the "Great Imitator".

Although widespread pain is common among all people who live with fibromyalgia, the symptoms and severity of them are diverse. Even the same symptoms will manifest themselves differently in each individual. Also, it is quite typical for fibromyalgia patients to experience numerous symptoms and medical issues that frequently occur together but do not have one specific cause.

Common symptoms that occur with fibromyalgia are chronic widespread pain in the body (varying from sharp shooting pains to deep aches and twitches in the muscles), pain or tenderness in the main tender points of the body when pressure is applied to them (located in the soft tissue on the back of the neck, shoulders, chest, elbows, hips, buttocks, lower back, shins, and knees), fatigue, stiffness, pain in the muscles and ligaments surrounding the jaw (called *temporomandibular joint disfunction*), tingling or numbness in hands and feet, sleep issues, impaired concentration and memory (often referred to as "fibro fog"), dizziness and balance impairment, as well as migraines and other kinds of chronic headaches.

Although there is no definitive cause known for fibro-myalgia, data suggests that it often occurs after an individual experiences a physical trauma, such as surgery, acute illness, or a car accident. It is believed that injury or trauma that some-how affects the central nervous system may act as a catalyst in the development of the syndrome. Studies indicate that genet-ics may play a factor in a person's likelihood for developing fibromyalgia. Gender also seems to have an effect, although it is unclear as to why. While the risk of developing fibromyalgia is not exclusive to one gender, far more women are diagnosed than men. Around 80 percent of the patients being treated for fibromyalgia are female. The majority of people who are diagnosed with the syndrome are women in their childbearing years, generally between the ages of 20 and 50 years old. Di-agnoses do occur among men of those same ages and elderly people, but not nearly as often. While it is not impossible for children to have fibromyalgia, it is rare.

Systemic Lupus Erythematosus (SLE)

Systemic lupus erythematosus is another form of arthritis that also is an *autoimmune disease*. SLE is the most common type of *lupus* and generally the type to which people are referring when they use the term "lupus." In the bodies of individuals with SLE, the immune system attacks healthy cells and tissues instead of defending the body against harmful organisms. Ev-ery organ system is affected by the disease and each system can be affected differently depending on the individual. This can cause damage to many parts of the body including the joints, skin, blood vessels, heart, lungs, kidneys, and brain.

People with systemic lupus erythematosus usually ex-perience symptoms such as extreme fatigue, pain or swelling in joints, muscle aches, skin rashes, fevers with no known cause, pale or purple fingers or toes, anemia, blood-clotting issues, mouth ulcers, swollen glands, dizziness, and head-aches. Systemic lupus erythematosus is also characterized by bouts of illness and remissions.

The causes of SLE are unknown but are believed to be linked to factors such as genetics, environmental factors, and hormones. Systemic lupus erythematosus has not been linked to a specific gene, but individuals who have lupus often also have family members with autoimmune conditions. While anyone can develop lupus, it most often occurs in women. It is also more common in women of African American, Native American, Hispanic, and Asian descents.

Gout

Gout is a common and painful form of arthritis that affects approximately 3 million adults in the United States. *Gout occurs when uric acid accumulates in your body. Uric acid* comes from the breakdown of substances called *purines* that are found in body tissues and in foods like dried beans and peas, liver, and anchovies. Typically, uric acid is dissolved in the blood, passed through the kidneys, and then excreted in urine. However, when that does not happen effectively and uric acid builds up, it creates needle-like crystals. When those crystals form in the joints, it causes extreme pain. Those same crystals can also cause kidney stones.

Gout often starts by attacking the person's big toe. It causes a sudden burning pain, stiffness, and swelling in the joint. It can also occur in the ankles, heels, knees, wrists, fingers, and elbows. These attacks can continue to happen over and over unless gout is controlled. Over time, if left untreated, gout attacks can harm the joints, tendons, and other tissues of the individual. In the beginning, gout attacks usually resolve themselves in a few days. Eventually, though, the gout attacks progress, happen more frequently, and last for longer periods.

The risks of developing gout have been linked to factors such as genetics, gender, and weight. Individuals are more likely to get gout if they have a family member who has it. Men are also much more likely to develop gout than women. Although gout can occur in people of any age, it is typically found in adults. Individuals who are overweight have an increased risk of getting gout because there is more tissue available to break down, which can lead to the production of excess uric acid. Eating too many foods rich in purines (like anchovies, asparagus, dried beans and peas, mackerel, mushrooms, sardines, and scallops) can also aggravate gout.

Did You Know?

• Although arthritis is often associated with growing older, almost two-thirds of the people diagnosed with arthritis are under the age of 65. Even children can be affected by some forms of arthritis.

• Arthritis is more common among women (24.3%) than men (18.7%) in every age group, and it affects members of all racial and ethnic groups.

• Arthritis is the nation's most common cause of disability. About 21 million American adults experience limitations from arthritis by the type or amount of work they can do or their ability to work at all.

Risk Factors

With over 100 different types of arthritis, the specific factors that affect the development of these conditions varies. However, the following risk factors have been shown to be collectively associated with an increased risk of developing arthritis. Risks can be either *modifiable*, meaning that measures can be taken to change them, or *non-modifiable*, which means they cannot be altered.

Non-Modifiable Risk Factors

Other Chronic Conditions: Arthritis often occurs simultaneously with other chronic conditions. Among the adults in the United States who have arthritis, nearly half (47%) report having at least one other disease or condition. Statistics also show that over half of adults with heart disease (57%) or diabetes (52%) and more than one-third with high blood pressure (44%) or obesity (36%) also have arthritis.

Age: The risk of developing most types of arthritis increases with age.

Gender: The majority of the types of arthritis are more commonly found in women. About 60% of all people diagnosed with some form of arthritis are women. Gout is more common in men.

Genetics: The presence of arthritis in the family has been shown to put individuals at higher risk of developing some form of arthritis. Genetics have also been linked to increasing the risk factors for -certain types of arthritis that are autoimmune disorders, such as rheumatoid arthritis and systemic lupus erythematosus.

Modifiable Risk Factors

Being Overweight or Obese: Excess weight can contribute to both the onset and progression of most types of arthritis.

Previous Joint Injuries: Suffering damage or injury to a joint may contribute to the development of arthritis in that area.

Infection: Infection in the body has the potential to cause the development of many types of arthritis.

National Organizations for More Information about Arthritis

There are several national organizations devoted to research-ing and informing the American public about arthritis. You can contact these organizations if you are interested in learn-ing more about arthritis, would like to ask specific questions, or need to request additional data related to the condition.

Arthritis Foundation
National Office
1330 W. Peachtree Street
Suite 100
Atlanta, GA 30309
Phone number: (404) 872-7100
Website: www.arthritis.org

Arthritis National Research Foundation
200 Oceangate, Suite 830
Long Beach, CA 90802
Phone number: (562) 437-6808
Toll-free phone number: (800) 588-2873
Website: www.curearthritis.org

Arthritis Research Institute of America
300 South Duncan Avenue
Suite 188
Clearwater, FL 33755
Toll-free phone number: (888) 554-2742 (ARIA)
Email: info@preventarthritis.org
Website: www.preventarthritis.org

National Institute of Arthritis and Musculoskeletal and
Skin Diseases (NIAMS)
Information Clearinghouse
National Institutes of Health
1 AMS Circle
Bethesda, MD 20892-3675
Phone number: (301) 495-4484
Toll-free phone number: (877) 22-NIAMS (877-226-4267)
Email: NIAMSinfo@mail.nih.gov
Website: www.niams.nih.gov

Common Treatments for Arthritis

Medications

The medications used to treat arthritis will differ depending
on the type of arthritis. Here are some of the medications
most commonly used by, or prescribed to, arthritis patients:

Corticosteroids: Like prednisone and cortisone, corticosteroids help to reduce inflammation and suppress the immune
system. They can be taken orally or be injected directly into
the site of the affected joint.

Disease-Modifying Antirheumatic Drugs (DMARDs):
DMARDs are commonly used to treat rheumatoid arthritis
because they slow or stop the immune system from attacking
the joints. Two types of DMARDs are methotrexate (Trexall)
and hydroxychloroquine (Plaquenil).

Analgesics: Analgesics help reduce pain, but do not address
inflammation. Examples include acetaminophen (like Tyle-
nol), tramadol (such as Ultram or Ryzolt) and narcotics that
contain hydrocodone (like Vicodin or Lortab) or oxycodone
(such as Percocet or Oxycontin).

Nonsteroidal Anti-Inflammatory Drugs (NSAIDs): Non-steroidal anti-inflammatory drugs decrease both pain and inflammation. Examples of over-the-counter NSAIDs are ibuprofen (Advil or Motrin IB) and naproxen (Aleve). Some types of NSAIDs are also available only by prescription. Some NSAIDs are also available in the form of creams or gels and can be rubbed directly on joints.

Using Physical Activity and Diet to Deal with Arthritis

Arthritis affects people in many different ways, so there is not a simple cure to the pain or symptoms associated with the disease, especially since there are so many various forms of arthritis. Also, the length of time the individual has been dealing with arthritis and how severely the illness is affecting the body also determine the types of treatment that may be necessary. Arthritis treatment focuses on relieving symptoms and improving joint function.

Physical activity is one treatment that seems to be encouraged among the types of arthritis. Exercises can improve range of motion and strengthen the muscles surrounding joints. Of course, the amount and types of exercise that will be most effective will depend on the form of arthritis and the extent of the damage it is causing to the body. In fact, physicians warn that inactivity could *harm* the health of most arthritis patients. Without regular physical activity, muscles grow weaker, joints become stiffer, balance problems worsen, and the individual's tolerance for pain decreases. Inactivity also increases the risks of cardiovascular disease and type 2 diabetes. Arthritis patients who are physically active usually enjoy better health, and experience improvements in pain, sleep, energy levels, and daily functioning.

David Borenstein, MD, President of the American College of Rheumatology and practicing rheumatologist says, "Many people with arthritis and rheumatic diseases suffer from joint pain and stiffness, which can cause a person to avoid exercise out of the fear of increasing their pain or causing injury. However, exercise, when properly planned and safely executed, can do just the opposite."

Experts also stress the importance of eating a well-balanced diet to deal naturally and effectively with arthritis. Not only will individuals receive vital nutrients from improving food choices, they will also be able to either maintain or achieve a healthy body weight. Carrying extra weight adds more pressure on the weight-bearing joints and exacerbates symptoms of arthritis. Many arthritis sufferers find that losing even a few pounds makes a positive difference in their quality of life.

Foods to Include in a Healthy Diet for Arthritis Patients

Overall, individuals with arthritis should try to aim for a diet that is high in fruits, vegetables, fish, nuts, legumes, and olive oil. Also, limiting or avoiding red meat, saturated fats, dairy, and sugar can help prevent arthritis and manage inflammation and pain related to arthritis.

Omega-3 Fatty Acids: Research shows that omega-3 fatty acids may prevent inflammation in the body and decrease symptoms associated with arthritis. While some foods increase levels of inflammation in the body, omega-3s actually work to decrease inflammation by suppressing the production of enzymes that erode cartilage. Omega-3 fatty acids are found in oily fish and fish oil supplements. Some of the best foods to consume for omega-3 fatty acids are salmon (wild, fresh, or canned), herring, sardines, rainbow trout, Pacific oysters, flaxseeds (ground and oil), chia seeds, and walnuts.

Cruciferous Vegetables: According to a study conducted by the Mayo Clinic, cruciferous vegetables like broccoli and cauliflower were shown to protect against the development of arthritis. Other good choices to add to your diet are cabbage, Brussels sprouts, kale, and bok choy.

Vitamin D: Studies have indicated that people who consumed more dietary vitamin D had a lower risk of developing some types of arthritis. Some foods like dairy products and bread may be fortified with vitamin D, however, they also may exacerbate arthritis inflammation and pain. Instead, try to increase your vitamin D intake from oily fish such as tuna, mackerel, cod, and sea bass. Also, get outside and soak up the best source of natural vitamin D—sunlight.

Olive Oil: Diets that contain high quantities of olive oil, like the Mediterranean style diets, have been shown to reduce pain and stiffness in individuals with arthritis. That is because olive oil contains anti-inflammatory properties that are attributed to its *oleic acid*—which contains polyphenols and omega-3 fatty acids, both of which are antioxidants. Olive oil also contains a natural compound called *oleocanthal* that blocks the same inflammatory pathways as medications often used to fight arthritis pain. For the highest antioxidant content, choose extra virgin olive oil.

Ginger: The Journal of Medicinal Food gives evidence to support the role of ginger as an anti-inflammatory and antioxidant. Try adding extra ginger to meals by adding sliced ginger to tea, grating fresh ginger over sautéed vegetables, or sprinkling ground ginger in batters. Be aware that ginger also acts as a blood thinner, which could interact with blood thinning medications.

Vitamin C: Vitamin C is one of the nutrients most responsible for the health of collagen, which is a major component of cartilage. Increased intake of vitamin C is also associated with reducing the risk of developing some forms of arthritis. Choose dietary sources of vitamin C rather than supplements because high doses of vitamin C supplements have been known to worsen symptoms of arthritis. Excellent sources of vitamin C-rich foods are bell peppers (yellow, red, orange, and green), oranges, guava, mangos, grapefruits, strawberries, pineapple, broccoli, cauliflower, and kidney beans.

Anthocyanidins: Anthocyanidins are potent antioxidants that produce the reddish pigment in foods like cherries, blackberries, raspberries, strawberries, grapes, and eggplant. A Harvard School of Public Health study showed that the anthocyanidins found in strawberries and other foods may help reduce inflammation associated with arthritis.

Green Tea: Green tea contains a natural antioxidant called *epigallocatechin-3-gallate* (EGCG) not found in black tea. Studies suggest that EGCG helps to prevent the production of certain inflammatory chemicals in the body, including the ones involved in arthritis. Preliminary research suggests that EGCG and other *catechins* (biologically active compounds found in plants that have potent antioxidants) in tea may stop cartilage from breaking down and possibly help to preserve joints longer.

Carotenes: Carotenoids are a group of powerful antioxidant nutrients contained in many fruits and vegetables. The most commonly known one is *beta carotene* (found in foods such as pumpkin, carrots, kale, butternut squash, cantaloupe, sweet potatoes, and spinach). Its sister carotenoid, *beta-cryptoxanthin,* may also decrease the risk of developing inflammation-related conditions like arthritis. Beta-cryptoxanthin is transformed into vitamin A in the body and may help prevent arthritis. Researchers have found that people who ate diets high in beta-cryptoxanthin were half as likely to develop a form of inflammatory arthritis as those who consumed low amounts. Excellent foods sources for beta cryptoxanthin are winter squash, pumpkin, persimmons, papaya, tangerines, sweet peppers, corn, collard greens, oranges, and apricots.

Below are some natural ways to add some other important vitamins and nutrients to your diet to boost and maintain your health:

Natural Sources of Vitamin B12:
• Clams
• Salmon
• Haddock
• Trout

Natural Sources of Vitamin A:
• Yellow vegetables (summer squash)
• Carrots
• Green leafy vegetables (such as kale, spinach, greens, and romaine lettuce)
• Fruits (such as cantaloupe, tomatoes, and apricots)

Natural Sources of Vitamin D:
• Tuna
• Liver oils
• Mackerel
• Cod
• Sea bass

Natural Sources of Calcium:
• Plain low-fat yogurt
• Sardines
• Salmon
• Any seafood that contains bones
• Turnip greens
• Spinach
• Kale
• Broccoli
• Nuts (such as almonds, Brazil nuts, and pecans)

Limit or Avoid These Inflammatory Foods

Trans Fats: Trans fats (which are also referred to as hydrogenated oils) are fats that are man-made in factories to prolong the shelf life of foods. The process makes vegetable oils more solid by adding hydrogen to liquid vegetable oil. Trans fats raise LDL (low-density lipoprotein) cholesterol level ("bad cholesterol") in the body and increases the risks of inflammation, heart disease, and other health issues. Trans fats are usually found in packaged and processed snack foods, crackers, cookies, shortenings, some margarine, fried foods, and baked goods like biscuits, pastries, and pizza dough.

Saturated Fats: Saturated fats are found primarily in animal products, like dairy (such as ice cream, butter, whole milk or 2-percent milk, and regular cheese) and meat products (like fatty beef, pork, and lamb; poultry skin; bacon; bologna; salami; and pepperoni). Foods that are high in saturated fat may increase the cholesterol in the blood, which can lead to clogged arteries that block blood flow to the brain and heart. Foods with a lot of saturated fat can also intensify inflammation (which is already associated with arthritis) and cause the immune system to become overactive. This leads to fatigue, joint pain, and damage to the blood vessels.

Fried Foods: High-fat foods like fried chicken, French fries, donuts, and other deep-fried items should be avoided by people who have arthritis. Fried foods, when eaten in excess, increase body fat and put extra stress on the joints. Also, some restaurants fry their foods in hydrogenated oils, which are the trans fats mentioned above. Instead of frying foods, try healthier options for cooking foods like grilling, steaming, roasting, and baking.

Refined Carbohydrates: Refined carbohydrates are found in foods baked with white flour, such as white bread, rolls, crackers, and most baked goods, as well as white rice and some cereals. They are manufactured by milling whole grains and removing the bran and germ, which are actually the two parts of the grain that have the most nutrients. Refined carbohydrates increase inflammation in the body and worsen the symptoms of arthritis. Limit foods made with refined grains and make healthier whole-grain choices like brown and wild rice, whole-wheat bread, whole-grain cereal, and whole-wheat pasta.

Simple Sugars: Simple sugars are found in foods like fruit juice, soft drinks, candy, and cookies. They are also refined carbohydrates and will dramatically increase blood-sugar levels. That, in turn, will initiate an inflammatory response in the body and make arthritis and its symptoms worse.

CHAPTER 2

THE BENEFITS OF YOGA

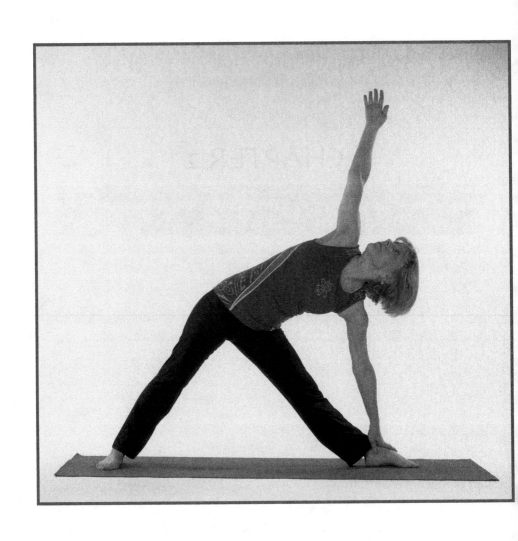

Physical activity is important for people with arthritis, although people with some forms or severe cases of arthritis may find it difficult to engage in more strenuous types of exercise. Yoga is one kind of exercise that is a wise choice for people with arthritis because it can be adapted and modified to meet the specific needs of the individual.

Yoga combines both *weight-bearing exercises* and *muscle-strengthening exercises*, making it a good option for people with arthritis. It is also a *low-impact* form of physical activity, so there is less danger of loss of balance or falls that may accompany more high-impact forms of exercise. Yoga combines both weight-bearing exercises and muscle-strengthening exercises, making it a wise choice for people with multiple sclerosis. It is also a low-impact form of physical activity, so there is less danger of loss of balance or falls that may accompany more high-impact forms of exercise.

The poses found in this book have been designed to accommodate various stages of the disease and include variations to help you tailor your yoga practice to your own level of mobility. If you are currently using a wheelchair, walker, or cane, you may find the chair variations helpful. However, always be sure to listen to your body and only do poses that feel safe and comfortable for you.

In addition to being a low-impact and customizable form of exercise, yoga also:

Offers relief from pain, stress and anxiety: Yoga is effective in alleviating pain, and reducing stress and anxiety, which can compromise systems in your body and affect functions like immunity and digestion. Yoga practices such as meditation help you focus on something other than what you are feeling. It also allows the entire body to relax and get the rest it needs to replenish itself.

Strengthens muscles and increases flexibility: Strong and flexible muscles boost the strength of the bones they surround and offer them added protection. Yoga provides a way to strengthen muscles and build flexibility without making your muscles too bulky. Strengthening the muscles, particularly those in the back and shoulders, also helps improve your posture. Yoga also helps release tension in the muscles.

Creates balance and coordination: Yoga is beneficial for individuals who have many forms of arthritis because it improves balance and coordination, which will make you more stable on your feet and help reduce the number of falls.

Stress Relievers: Breathing, Meditation, and Visual Imagery

The manner in which you respond to stress may exacerbate your existing symptoms or induce an arthritis attack. For instance, stress often prompts more instances of sleep problems, overeating, abuse of alcohol and illicit drugs, and smoking.

A Breathing Exercise: The Gateway to Daily Meditation

Focusing on the breath is one of the most common and fundamental techniques for accessing the *meditative state*. Breath is a deep rhythm of the body that connects us intimately with the world around us. Learn these steps, and then practice them as a regular breathing exercise.

Close your eyes, breathe deeply and regularly, and observe your breath as it flows in through the nose and out of the mouth. Give your full attention to the breath as it comes in and goes out. Store your breath in the belly, not the chest, between inhales and exhales. Whenever you find your attention wandering away from your breath, gently pull it back to the rising and falling of the breath via the belly.

Inhale through your nose slowly and deeply, feeling the

lower chest and abdomen inflate like a balloon. Hold for five seconds. Exhale deeply, deflating the lower chest and abdomen like an emptying balloon. Hold for five seconds. Do this five times, and then allow your breathing to return to a normal rhythm.

You will begin to feel a change come over your entire body. Gradually you will become less aware of your breathing, but not captured in your stream of consciousness. Consciousness is encouraged on the whole, but we often are too alert and hyper-stimulated via television, caffeine, and family life, just to name a few. By breathing for five minutes daily, you will become more centered inward. You will just live "in the moment," in your own skin.

Benefits of a simple breathing exercise throughout the day include:

• Calming
• "Re-centering" one's thoughts
• Increase in the flow of blood that carries oxygen through the body and improved efficiency of exhaling and ridding the body of carbon dioxide
• Decreased levels of fatigue later in the day, legs won't feel "heavy"

Increasing oxygenated blood via deep breathing can decrease muscle pains, especially in the *postural muscles* (back and neck muscles), and can also help counteract chronic stressors such as sitting or standing in static positions for extended periods of time.

Deep Breathing
Practice deep breathing as a form of relaxation before bed. Slow, deep breathing is an excellent way to slow the heart rate and contemplate the day's events. Focus on breathing in through the nose and out through the mouth.

Simple Stress Reliever

Looking for a simple, healthy way to help get through the day? Try breathing exercises—a wonderfully effective way to reduce stress, maintain focus, and feel energized. Exhaling completely is one breathing exercise to try—it can promote deeper breathing and better health.

Give it a try: Simply take a deep breath, let it out effortlessly, and then squeeze out a little more. Doing this regularly will help build up the muscles between your ribs, and your exhalations will soon become deeper and longer. Start by practicing this exhalation exercise consciously, and before long it will become a healthy, unconscious habit.

Meditation Tips for Beginners

Yoga offers meditation and controlled breathing techniques that are used effectively to manage the pain associated with arthritis and refocus your thoughts. Meditating for only a few minutes each day can help. Here are a few quick tips for meditation beginners:

• Take the time to stretch out first. Loosening muscles and tendons before beginning allows you to sit or lie more comfortably.
• Make it a formal practice by setting aside a specific time and place to devote to your meditation.
• Focus on the breathing. Slowing your breathing helps your mind and body to relax and prepare for meditation.
• Meditate in the morning. It is usually quieter in the morning, and your mind has not yet had the chance to get cluttered. It will also help work out any kinks in your body from sleeping. And it's always great to start your day with focus!
• Find a time and place to meditate where you will not be disturbed.
• Enlist the help of instructional videos or calming music if they help you relax more.

• Light a candle and use it as a focal point, instead of closing your eyes. Focusing on the light causes you to strengthen your attention.

• Be aware of your body and how it feels in both its normal and relaxed states, and embrace the differences.

• Experiment with different types of meditation and different positions. You won't know which methods works best for you until you try them.

• Have a purpose behind your meditation, such as pain management or feeling more focused on a specific issue you must deal with.

• Push aside feeling of doubt, frustration, and stress about whether or not you are doing it right. It is counterproductive to your meditation.

• Relax and relish in your mind's incredible ability to focus and care for your body through meditation.

• Remember your meditation and breathing techniques throughout the day. A few well-placed cleansing breaths will do wonders for your mind and body.

Some of the most commonly recommended yoga poses for individuals with arthritis can be found in this book, including:

Mountain
Warrior I
Warrior II
Warrior III
Child
Seated Twist
Tree
Triangle
Corpse
Hero
Downward-Facing Dog

CHAPTER 3

SAFETY PRECAUTIONS

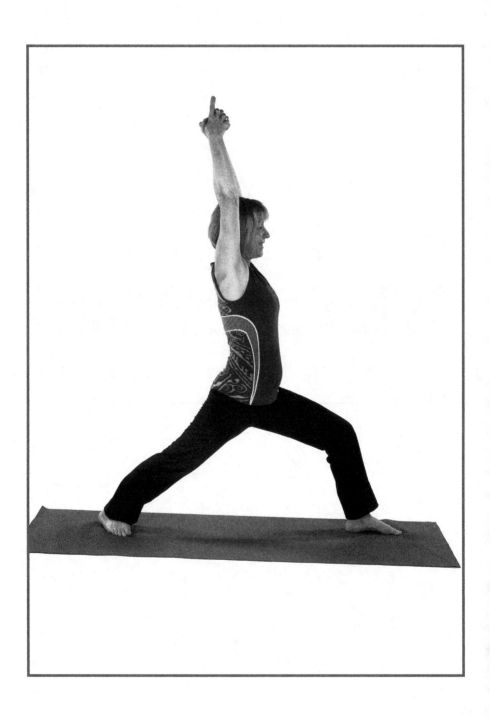

Even though an active lifestyle is healthy and encouraged, there are some exercises that may actually cause more harm than good. If you have arthritis, it is best to avoid *overexerting* yourself with exercise or physical activity because some symptoms may become exacerbated by pushing too hard. Yoga is one beneficial practice that can be safely modified to aid people who have arthritis pain. It's important to remember that, as your body changes and matures, the way you practice yoga must also change. Approach your yoga practice with gentleness and acceptance of the body you have now, and allow it to work safely for you.

Follow these guidelines to ensure safety when practicing yoga exercises for arthritis:

• It is always recommended that you talk to your doctor before starting an exercise program.
• Once you have the approval of your doctor, start the exercise program and ease into the more difficult moves. These gentle yoga exercises are intended to strengthen your body and relieve some of the symptoms associated with your arthritis, not aggravate them.
• If a pose seems too difficult or is painful in any way, try the variation pose instead.
• If you are currently using a wheelchair, walker, or cane, try the chair variations of the poses as these have been designed specifically for individuals with restricted mobility.
• If you are new to yoga, you may find it best to start by holding the poses for only a few long, deep breaths. As you progress and feel more comfortable, you can begin to hold the poses for longer.
• Concentrate more on maintaining proper alignment while doing your yoga exercises and focus less on pushing over your limits. Recognize your limitations and respect them. Trying to surpass them may inflict unnecessary pain or risk of injury.
• Since everyone has varying degrees of flexibility and pain associated with arthritis and its symptoms, it is important not to gauge your level of difficulty against someone else's. Practice

the yoga exercises to the degree that you can perform them comfortably and safely for your own body.

• There are no specific yoga postures that must be avoided by individuals with arthritis, but please use wisdom and listen to your body. If any of the yoga moves cause you pain or intensify your arthritis symptoms, stop immediately. Generally, you will notice pain if you are going too far with the pose, but sometimes the effects may not be felt until the next day. Remember to be gentle with your yoga practice, especially when you are just beginning. If you do not experience any pain after a few days, you may decide to gradually increase the intensity of your yoga poses.

Yoga Adapted for Practice with a Wheelchair

Some people with more severe arthritis may find it difficult to move around and will need the help of a mobility aid, like a wheelchair. Even if your arthritis has caused you to need a wheelchair, you can still practice yoga!

When practicing yoga from a wheelchair, there are a few things to keep in mind. First, it is important to understand that wheelchair confinement significantly atrophies the muscles in the back and abdomen. Without the support of these core muscles, the spine slackens and begins to bend forward. This compresses the abdomen, rib cage, and lungs, which makes deep breathing nearly impossible. In turn, shallow breathing restricts the flow of oxygen and blood circulation, both of which exacerbate physical ailments and mobility. As a result, it is important to gradually strengthen these core muscles in working towards achieving the appropriate posture for these yoga poses. The quality of your posture directly correlates with the benefits you will receive from yoga.

Before beginning any poses in your wheelchair, be sure to consult your doctor. It is also important that you have the assistance of a caregiver, especially if you are a beginner. Also, remember that yoga should stimulate your muscles, but your practice should never cause pain. If you experience pain during a pose, stop immediately.

Remember to breathe deeply while holding each pose (for breathing advice, see page 24). Many of the seated poses in this book can be also practiced in a wheelchair.

Here are some more wheelchair options for some of the other poses:

Forward Bend (see page 84)

Begin by following the directions for seated Mountain pose (see page 38). Hold onto your wheelchair just below the seat or place your hands on top of your thighs for support. As you inhale, lengthen through your spine. As you exhale, bend forward while maintaining the length in your spine. Hold this pose for three to five breaths and continue to breathe deeply.

Warrior I (see page 42)

With your feet directly below your knees, sit upright in your wheelchair. Do not lean on your chair's back support. Have an assistant place a chair in front of you. The seat should be facing away from you. Shift your hips to the left; slightly raise left buttocks off the seat.

Gradually draw your left leg back. Use your hand to position your left leg, if necessary. Slowly begin to drop your left knee forward and bring your knee to the ground. Be sure to keep your left knee in line with your hip. If your knee does not reach the ground, have an assistant place a folded blanket under your knee.

Place your palms on the top of the chair. Inhale and extend through your back and ribcage. If possible, raise your arms above the head and interlock your fingers. Hold for three to five breaths. Repeat on the other side.

Warrior II (see page 44)

Sit forward while still remaining comfortable and maintaining balance. With your thighs separated and feet flat on the floor, bend your left knee at a 90-degree angle. Then fully straighten your right leg. On your next inhalation, bring your arms into the "T" position. Focus your eyes on the fingertips of your left hand. Hold for five breaths. Repeat on the other side.

Seated Twist (see page 78)

Sitting upright, gently twist to the right and take your left hand over to the right side of the wheelchair. Hold onto the arm or side of the wheelchair to help twist to the right. Coming back to center, sit upright and then twist gently to the left, bringing your right hand over to the left side of the wheelchair and gently twist to the left.

Downward-Facing Dog (see page 62)

Press the back of your wheelchair against a sturdy wall. Have an assistant place a folding chair about two feet away, facing your wheelchair. You may fasten your safety belt as an extra precaution.

With your feet directly under knees, place your hands on the seat of the folding chair. As you inhale, raise the top of your head, extending through your spine. Be sure to keep your chin parallel to the floor. Drop your shoulders downward. On the next exhale, press the chair forward to align your ears with your shoulders as you press your hips back and heels down. Continue to press your palms firmly into the seat for three to five breaths. Then return to an upright position.

This pose can also be done facing a wall by pressing your palms and forehead to the wall instead of the chair.

Child (see page 92)

Have an assistant place a folding chair in front of your wheelchair. Be sure that the seat is facing you. Place a rolled-up mat on the seat of the chair. The place a bolster cushion parallel to you, with one end resting on your lap and the other end resting on the seat of the chair. Add a folded blanket to rest your forehead on. Lean forward and rest your head on the blanket. No pressure should be on your nose. You can either rest your arms on the seat of the chair or try crossing them above your head. Close your eyes and relax your face and body. Maintain smooth, even breathing, and try to remain focused on your breath.

CHAPTER 4

THE POSES

MOUNTAIN

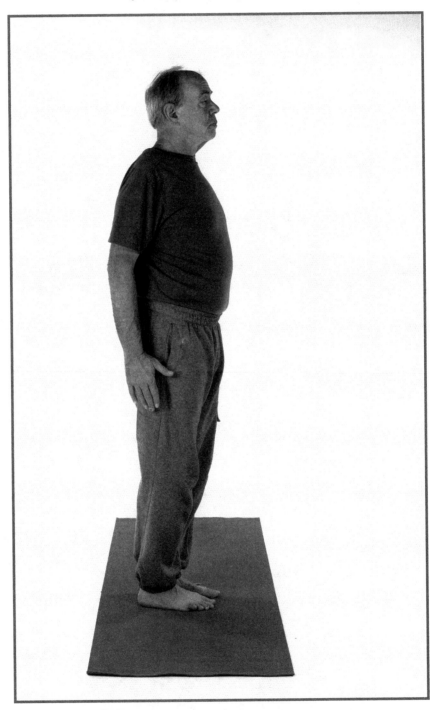

MODIFICATION

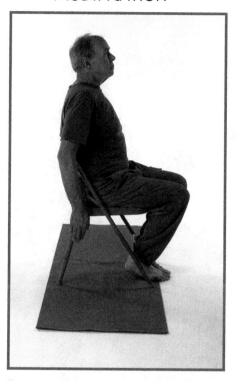

Stand with your big toes touching. Roll your shoulders up, back, and down—this movement places your shoulder blades on your back. Try to find your balance over the arches of your feet by rocking back and forth from the balls of your feet to the heels. Then build your body up from your feet and through your calves, pulling your kneecaps up, tightening your thighs, and tucking your tailbone under. Your chin should be centered with your chest. Exhale and pull up on your pelvic floor. On the next exhale, pull your stomach up and back (this will create strength in your abdominals). This "lock" in the abdominals should be used in all standing postures.

For the chair variation, sit upright in a chair with your legs and feet together and your arms at your sides. Roll your shoulders up, back, and down, then follow the directions to create a "lock" in your abdominals.

HANDS UNDER TOES

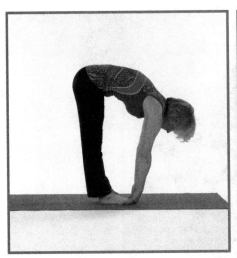 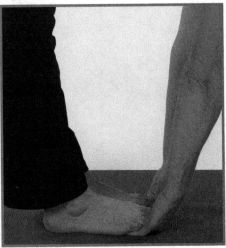

Start with your feet together in Mountain pose (see page 38). On the inhale, sweep your arms widely up and back. On the exhale, swan-dive down and bring your fingers under your toes, bending your knees as much as needed. On the inhale, raise your head and chest, keeping your fingers in place. On the exhale, lower your head. Repeat four to five times.

Note: This pose should be done from the hips, not the waist. As always, use caution and be sure to "listen" to your body—if the pose becomes too difficult, stop or switch to a more gentle variation.

LATERAL STRETCH

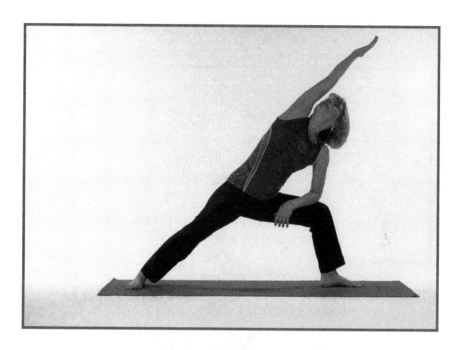

Start with your feet together in Mountain pose (see page 38) in the middle of the mat. Take a wide-legged stance and turn your right foot out 90 degrees. On the exhale, bend your right knee, keeping the outside of your left foot on the floor. On the next exhale, drop your right forearm to your thigh and, on the inhale, raise your left arm up. On the next exhale, stretch your left arm over your head while stretching from your left foot through your leg, hips, ribs and out from the fingertips of your left hand. With your palm facing down, turn your head to look at your palm—this keeps your neck in line with your spine. Hold for five breaths and repeat on the left side. As you gain strength in your legs, you may try this by using a block on the outside of your right foot. On the exhale, place your right hand down to the block and proceed as before. This pose may also be done with a chair by straddling the chair, positioning your legs in Warrior II (see page 44) and then proceeding with the arm movements.

WARRIOR I

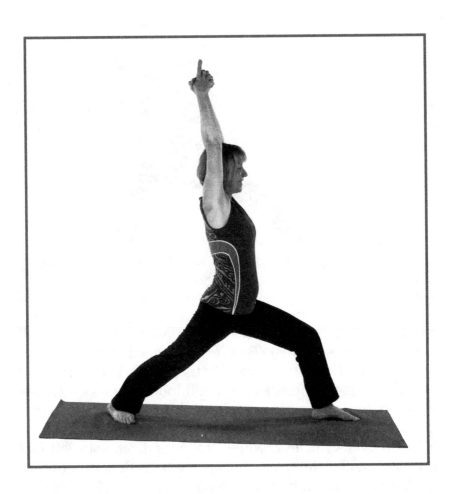

Start with your feet together in Mountain pose (see page 38). Take a wide-legged stance and turn your right foot out 90 degrees. Turn to face over your right foot with your shoulders and your hips. On the exhale, bend your right knee. On the inhale, raise your arms over your head and interlock your fingers. For increased intensity (not pictured), look up at your hands and hold for five breaths. Repeat on the left side.

MODIFICATION

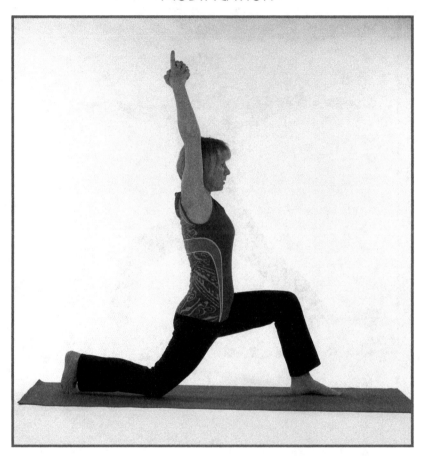

If this seems difficult, you may drop your back knee to the floor until you gain balance and strength.

WARRIOR II

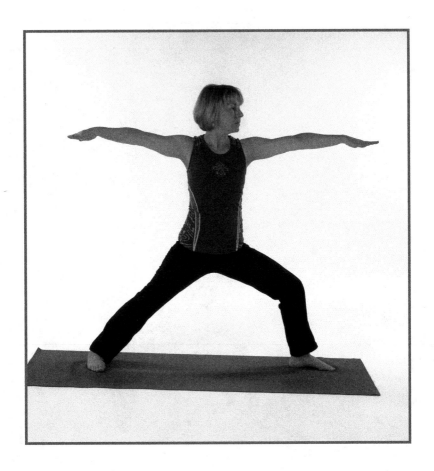

Start with your feet together in Mountain pose (see page 38). Take a wide-legged stance and, on the exhale, turn your left foot out 90 degrees, keeping your hips and shoulders facing forward. On the inhale, raise your arms into a 'T' position. On the next exhale, bend your left knee over your ankle. Your weight should be on the outside of your right foot as you pull up in your inner right thigh. Your focal point will be at the fingertips of your left hand. Hold for five breaths. Repeat on the other side.

MODIFICATION

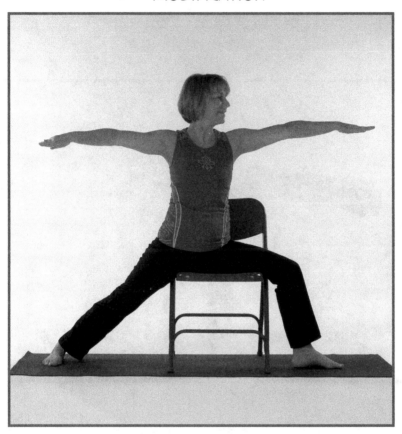

For the chair variation, sit on a chair and come to a straddle position. Bend your left knee and turn your left foot out 90 degrees. Extend your right leg out straight. On the inhale, raise your arms up and hold for five breaths.

WARRIOR III

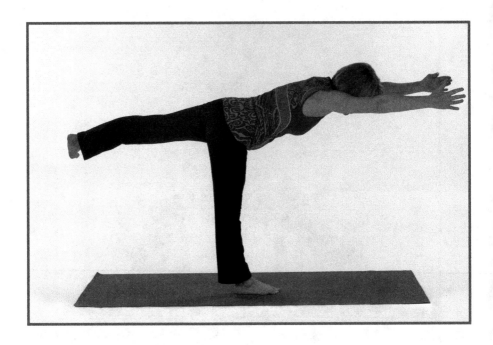

Start with your feet together, placing your weight on your left foot. On the inhale, raise your arms shoulder-width over your head. On the exhale, come forward with your torso and raise your right leg behind, keeping your hips parallel. Tighten your left leg and your abdominal muscles to hold your body up. Work up to five breaths. Repeat on the left side.

MODIFICATION

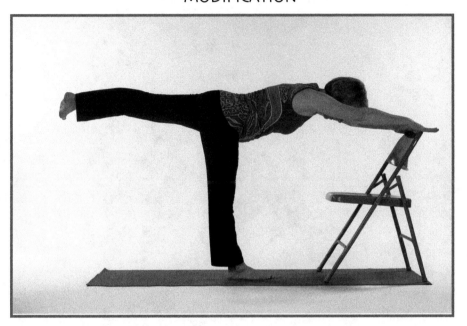

If this seems difficult, the pose can also be performed with your hands against the wall or on a chair, as shown.

TRIANGLE

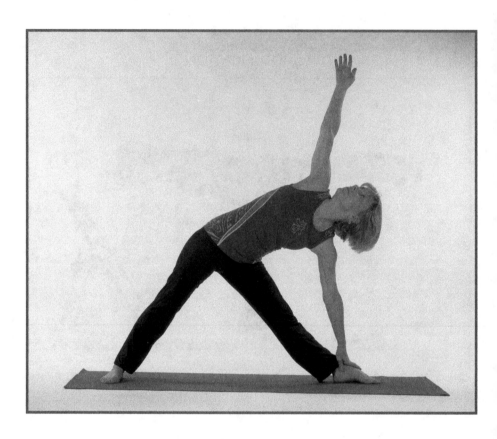

Start with your feet together in Mountain pose (see page 38) in the middle of the mat. Take a wide-legged stance and turn your right foot out 90 degrees. On the inhale, raise your arms into a 'T' position, extending them out from your shoulders. On the exhale, reach your right arm up, out, and down while pulling in on your right hip (this is a lunge movement to the right). Bring your right hand to rest on your leg wherever it goes easily (this means your hand may be as high as your knee since you are aiming for alignment of your shoulder over your leg).

MODIFICATION

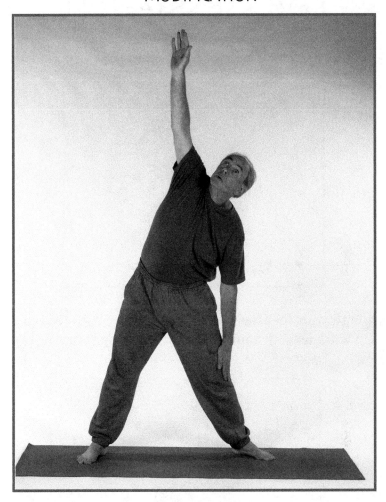

On the next breath, reach your left arm up towards the ceiling, keeping both legs straight (a block may be used here by placing it on the outside of your right foot and extending out and then down to the block). Try to turn your head to look up at your left hand, this will keep you neck in line with the spine. Hold for five breaths.

REVERSE TRIANGLE

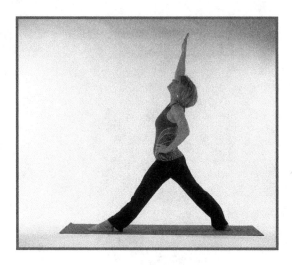

Start with your feet together in Mountain pose (see page 38). Take a wide-legged stance and turn your right foot out 90 degrees.

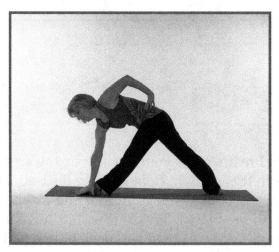

Place the block (if using) on the outside of your right foot and then turn your body to face over your right foot with both hips and shoulders facing right. Place your right hand on your hip.

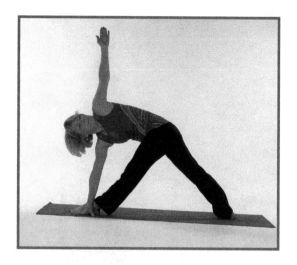

On the inhale, raise your left arm up and back, stretching back. On the exhale, start the twist as you come forward, placing your left hand to your knee, the block, or the floor. Hold for five breaths. For increased intensity, raise your right arm towards the ceiling while looking up at your hand.

When using the block, remember that it has three heights and beginners should start with the highest level.

Note: This pose should be done from the hips, not the waist. As always, use caution and be sure to "listen" to the body—if the pose becomes too difficult, stop or switch to a more gentle variation.

TREE

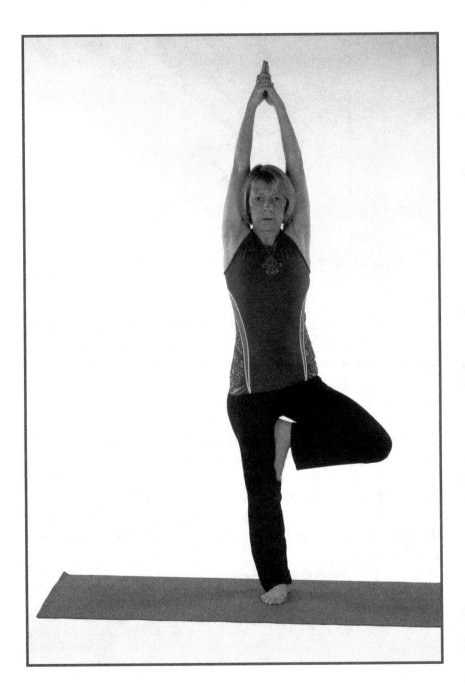

MODIFICATION 1

MODIFICATION 2

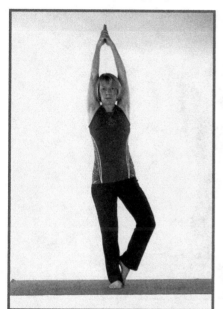

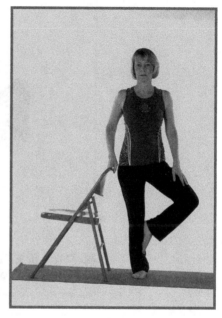

Start with your feet together in Mountain pose (see page 38). Shift your weight to your right leg and raise your left leg, placing the sole of your left foot on the inside of your right leg. Try to place your left foot as high as possible on your right leg, taking care not to place it on the inside of your knee (you may use a chair, as shown, or the wall to hold on to in the beginning). Bring your hands together in the center of your chest, with your hands in prayer position. Hold for five breaths. For increased intensity, raise your arms overhead, keeping your hands together and bringing your arms as close to your ears as possible.

STANDING LEG LIFT

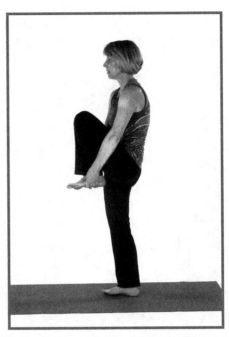

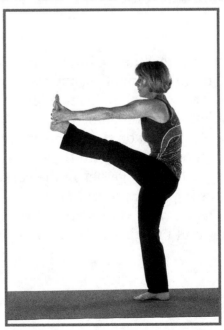

MODIFICATION 1

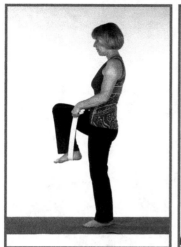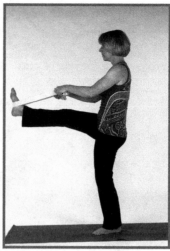

MODIFICATION 2

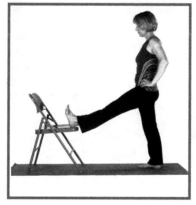

Start with your feet together in Mountain pose (see page 38), placing your weight on your left leg. Bend your right knee and wrap a strap under your right foot. Hold the strap in your right hand and straighten your right leg out in front of your body. For increased intensity (not pictured), bring your right leg out to the right and use your left arm for balance by placing it out to the left. Work up to five or six breaths. Repeat on the other side. This may also be done using a chair by placing your foot on the chair. As you gain balance and strength, move the strap as described. Once this becomes easy to perform with the strap, try bending your knee and grabbing your foot in your hands, then extend out.

DANCING SHIVA

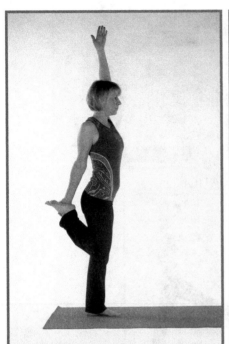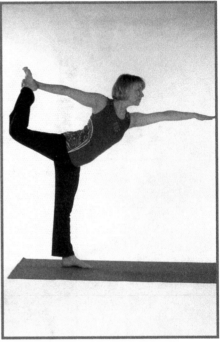

Start with your feet together in Mountain pose (see page 38).
Shift your weight to your right leg and raise your left leg, bending at the knee. Bring your left foot up behind you and grab
your foot with your palm facing up in the inside of your foot.
You may hold here or, for increased intensity, raise your right
arm straight up and on the exhale, bring your arm forward
then extend your left leg back and up. Work up to five breaths.
Repeat on the left side.

MODIFICATION

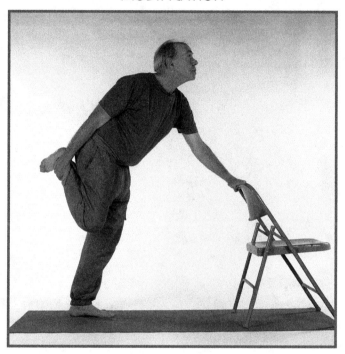

For the chair variation, place a chair arms-length in front of your body and proceed as described, placing your hand on the back of the chair for balance.

HALF MOON

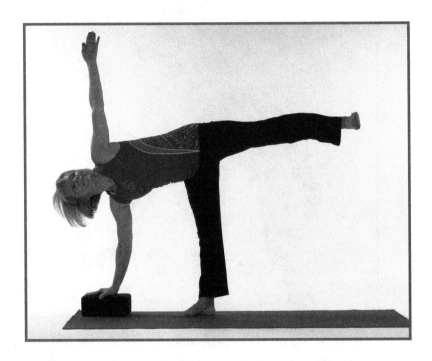

Beginners should use a block for this pose, placing the block by your right foot. Begin with your feet together in Mountain pose (see page 38) in the middle of the mat. Take a wide-legged stance, turn your right foot out 90 degrees, and bend your right knee so that your chest is resting on your right thigh. Place the block in your hand and bring it at least six inches in front of your right foot, keeping it in line with your baby toe. On the inhale, straighten your right leg while lifting your left. Keep your weight in your right leg and hand. Tighten your abdominals and both legs (the block has three levels, so start at the highest level and as you gain strength and balance use the lower levels).

MODIFICATION

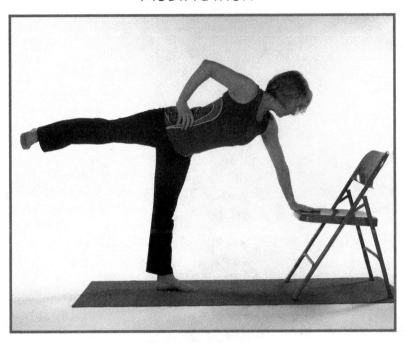

Place your left hand on your waist and work up to five full breaths. As this pose becomes easier, you may wish to increase the intensity by raising your left arm up towards the ceiling while turning your head to look up at your hand. You may also use a different height on the block, working towards the goal of placing your hand on the floor. Repeat on the left side.

For the chair variation, place a chair six to ten inches away from your right foot. In a wide-legged stance, proceed as described above, placing your hand on the chair for balance.

EAGLE

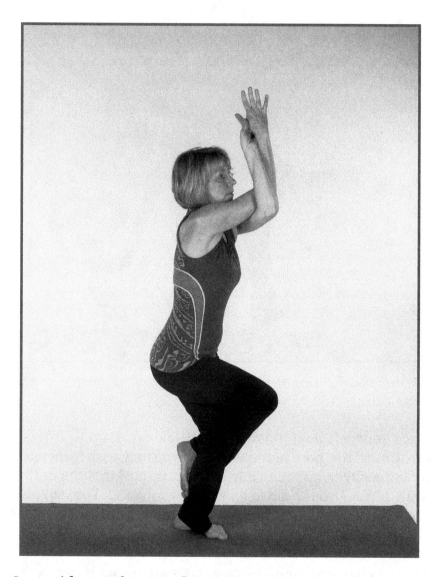

Start with your feet together in Mountain pose (see page 38).
Put your weight in your left foot, bring your right arm on top
of the left, and intertwine the arms to bring the hands together. Bend your left leg and wrap your right leg around your left
as you bring your hands either under your chin or raise them.
Hold for 5 breaths.

CAT AND DOG

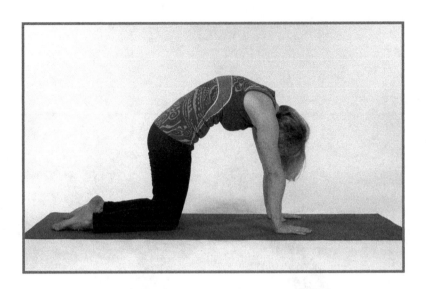

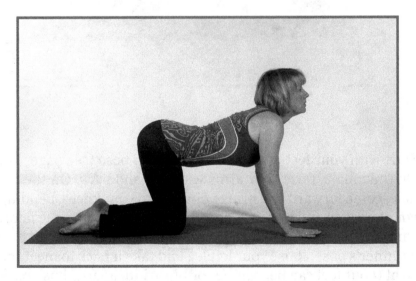

Start on all fours with your hands under your shoulders and your knees under your hips. On the exhale, round your back up to arch like a cat and bring your hips forward. Bring your chin to your chest. On the inhale, drop your belly and raise your head, pushing your sitting bones back and up. Repeat four to five times with the breath.

DOWNWARD-FACING DOG

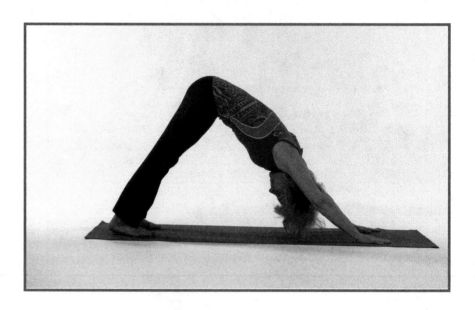

Start with your feet together in Mountain pose (see page 38).
On the inhale, raise your arms wide, up and back. On the exhale, come forward and bring your face to your knees, bending
your knees as much as needed to bring your palms to the floor.
On the exhale, raise your right leg and place it behind you into
a runner's pose. Raise your left leg and take it back to meet the
right (your feet can be together or hip-width apart). Push back
through your hands and arms until you are in an inverted 'V'
position. Your head should be between your arms, with your
hips pushing up and heels pushing down. Your weight will be
in your feet, palms, and index fingers. Hold for five breaths.
To come up, step forward.

MODIFICATION

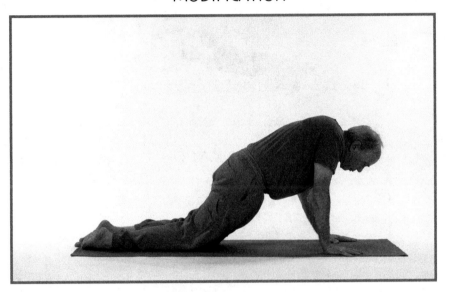

This may also be done by starting in a kneeling position on your hands and knees (in a tabletop position), then curling your toes under and pushing back into an inverted 'V' position.

UPWARD-FACING DOG

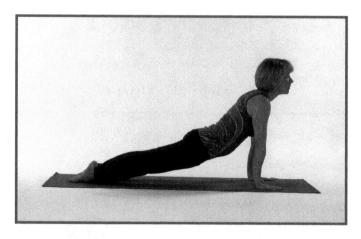

MODIFICATION

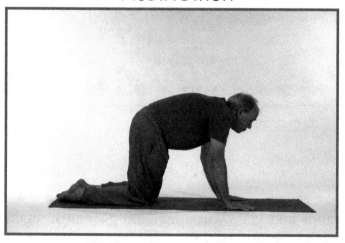

Start by lying on the mat on your stomach, with your forehead on the floor. Bring your hands under your shoulders, keeping your elbows close to your body and your legs and feet together. On the inhale, push up with your arms, raise your head, then roll your shoulders up and back, while pushing against your hands. Rising up, lift your hips and thighs off the mat so that your weight is on the top of your feet and in your hands. If this is difficult, you can raise up to your knees, working up to rising to your feet. Work up to five breaths.

SPHINX

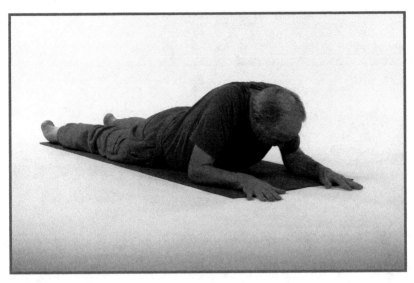

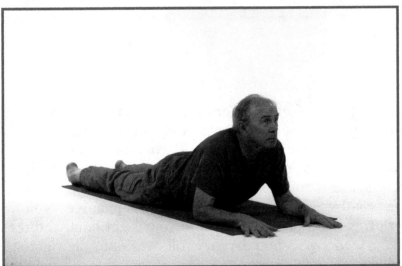

Lie on your stomach and bring your forehead to the floor. With your legs and feet together, bring your arms up and position your elbows under your shoulders, keeping your forearms stretched out in front of your torso. On the inhale, rise up onto your elbows and hold for five breaths or more. Come down, take a breath or two, and then rise back up for another five breaths.

PLANK

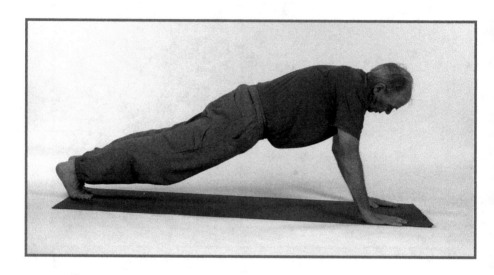

Start with your feet together in Mountain pose (see page 38).
On the inhale, sweep your arms up. On the exhale, bend forward and swan-dive down. Bend your knees as needed to
place your hands on the floor under your shoulders. Step your
feet back and create a straight line with your body. Hold for
five breaths. For increased intensity (not pictured), you may
perform a side plank. Make sure your right hand is directly
under your right shoulder and roll over onto the right side,
trying to stack your feet one on top of the other. You can then
also try to raise your left arm or keep it at your waist. Come
back to the center plank and roll onto the left side (if performing the side plank).

MODIFICATION

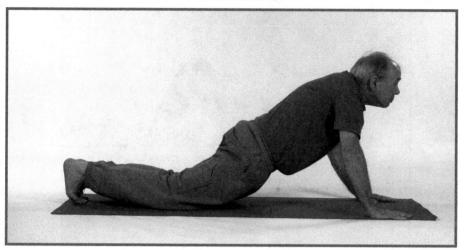

For beginners, start on your hands and knees (in a tabletop position) and step one foot back at a time until you can hold the pose with both feet back.

BOAT

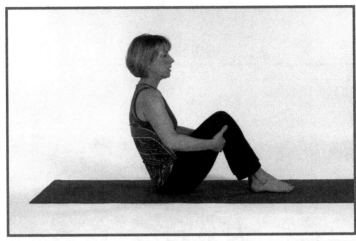

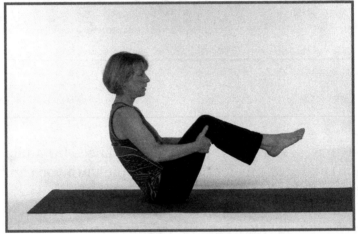

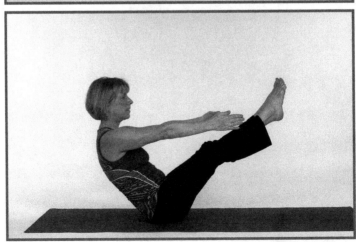

MODIFICATION

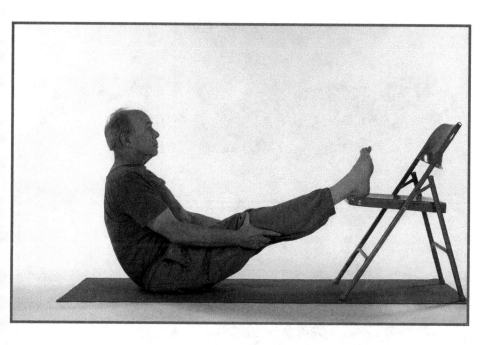

Come to a sitting staff position (sit on the mat with your back straight and your legs out in front of you). Bend your knees and bring the soles of your feet to the floor as you grab behind your knees. Rock back, holding your legs until your feet come off the floor. Try to straighten your legs and hold (you may continue to hold your legs until your abdominal muscles become strong enough to hold your body up). For increased intensity, stretch your arms out along the sides of your legs and hold for five or more breaths.

For the chair variation, place a chair in front of you and bring your feet onto the edge of the chair, proceeding as described above.

LOCUST

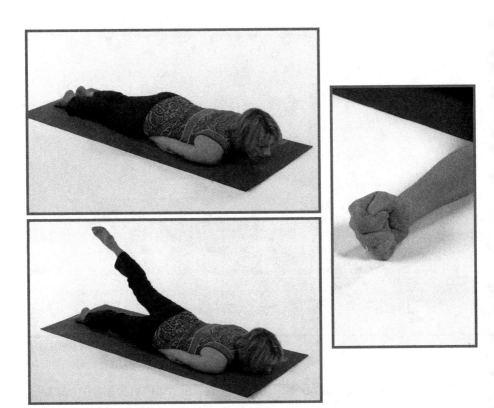

Lie on your stomach with your chin on the floor and your legs and feet together. Make a fist with your hand by wrapping your fingers around your thumbs. Bring your hands under your body at your groin. On the inhale, raise your left leg and hold for up to five breaths. Lower your leg and, on the next inhale, raise your right leg and hold, keeping your chin on the floor.

Variation 1 (not pictured): Bring your hands under your body with your palms down and pinkies touching. Repeat the sequence.

MODIFICATION

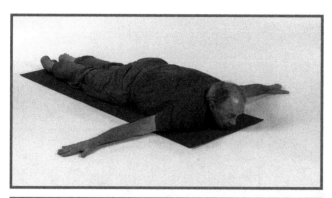

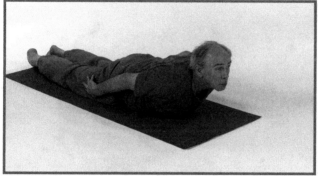

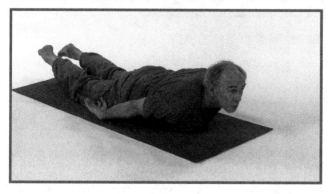

Variation 2: Bring your arms out in a 'T' position and, on the inhale, sweep them back and raise your head and chest. Raise your legs.

MODIFICATION

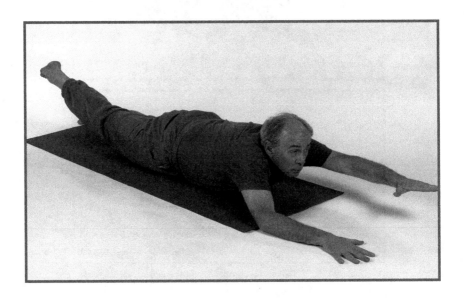

Variation 3: Bring your arms out in front of your body and raise your left arm and right leg, hold, then lower. Raise your right arm and left leg, hold, then lower. Finally, raise both arms and both legs (not pictured), hold, then lower.

MODIFICATION

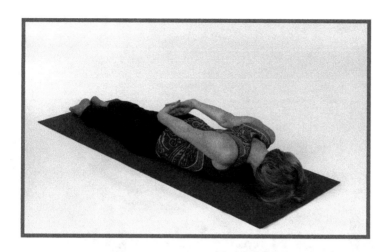

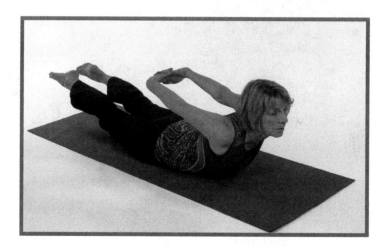

Variation 4: Bring your hands behind your back and interlock your fingers. On the inhale, raise your head, chest, and arms. Then raise your legs, hold, and breathe.

BOW

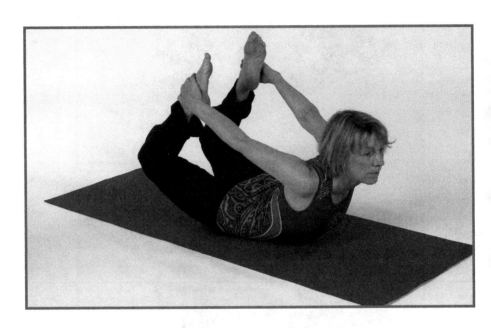

Lie face down with your forehead on the floor. Bend your knees and bring your feet towards your head, reaching back for your feet (a strap can be used to modify this pose, not pictured). On the inhale, raise your head and chest, then raise your legs, trying to bring your thighs off the floor. Work up to holding for five to six breaths, then repeat.

MODIFICATION

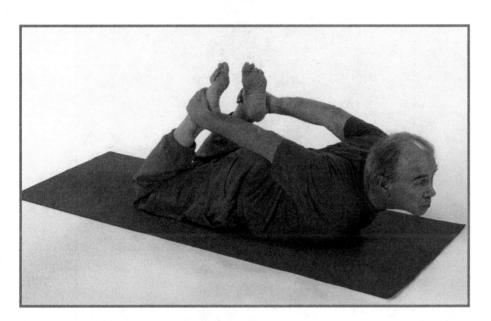

If you are unable to raise your thighs all the way, you can perform the poses as described, while keeping your thighs on the
mat.

Note: As always, use caution and be sure to "listen" to your
body—if the pose becomes too difficult, stop or switch to a
more gentle variation.

FULL SQUAT

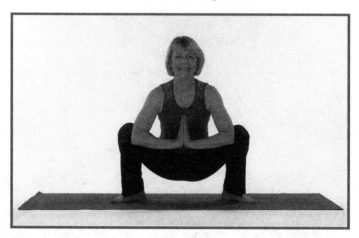

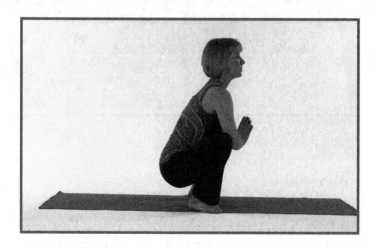

Start with your feet a little more than hip-width apart and your toes pointing out (your feet can be out as far as the edge of the mat). Bring your hands together in prayer position and bend your knees, coming down as far as you can while keeping the soles of your feet on the ground. Work up to five breaths. To come up, place your hands on the floor and straighten your legs, then slowly roll your spine up.

UPWARD-FACING BENT LEG

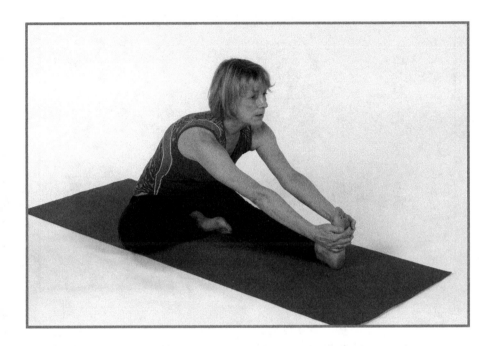

Sit tall and straight on the mat with both legs out in front of you, keeping your feet together. Bring your right leg in, placing the sole of your right foot against the inside of your left thigh. On the inhale, bring your arms overhead and look up at your hands. On the exhale, bend from your hips into a forward bend over your left leg, and reach as close to your foot as possible. Look at the horizon and hold for 5 breaths, then switch legs, and finish by performing the pose with both legs out (not pictured).

Note: As always, use caution and be sure to "listen" to your body—if the pose becomes too difficult, stop or switch to a more gentle variation.

SEATED TWIST

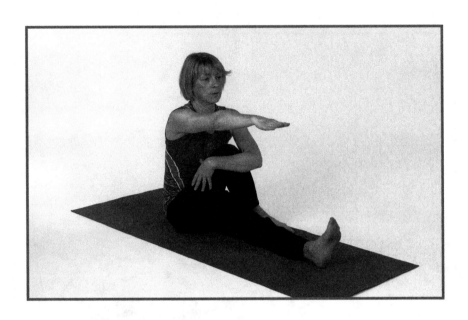

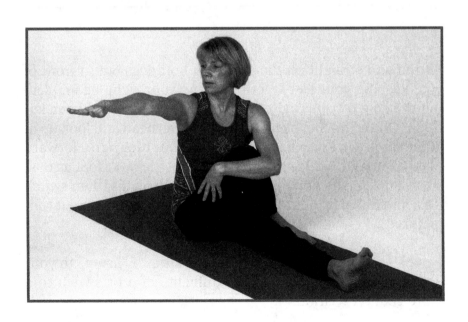

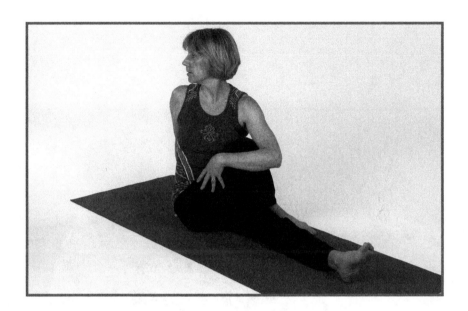

Sit with your legs together and extended straight out. Bring your right leg up and cross it over your left leg, placing the sole of your right foot on the outside of your left thigh. Hold your right knee with your left arm, raising your right arm straight out in front of your body. On the exhale, turn to your right with your arm extended and follow with your head, placing your hand on the floor behind your back. Hold for five breaths and slowly release by first turning your head forward, then releasing your leg. Repeat on the other side.

Note: Be sure to only twist as far as is comfortable, being careful not to twist your neck too far.

RECLINED SPINAL TWIST

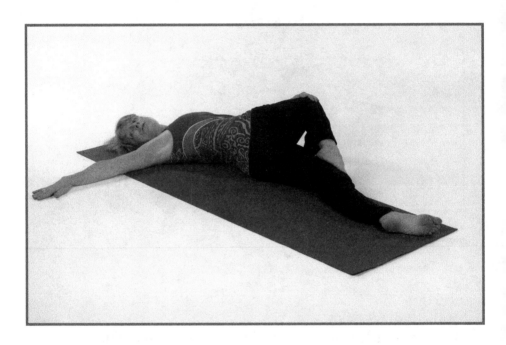

Lie on your back with your legs and feet together. Bring your right foot up and place the sole on your left thigh. Place your right arm out into a 'T' position and position your left hand on the outside of your right knee. On the exhale, twist to the left with your knee and look to the right with your head. Twist until you feel resistance and then hold for five breaths. Repeat on the other side.

MODIFICATION

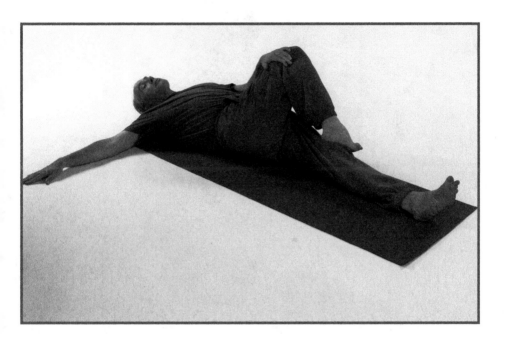

If you are unable to twist all the way to the left, you can twist halfway or as far as is comfortable for you.

HERO

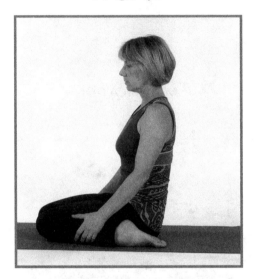

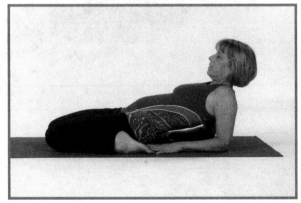

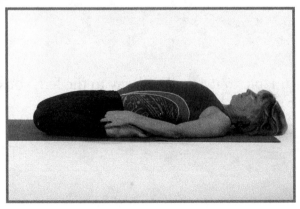

MODIFICATION

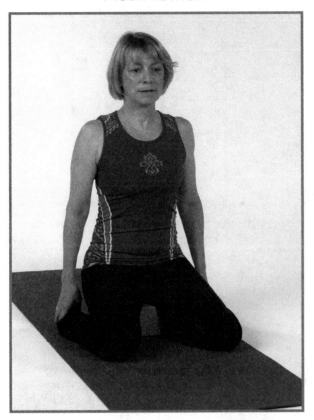

Come onto your knees. Try to sit back between your legs. If this is difficult, use a blanket under your knees or rest your sitting bone on a block (start by using the highest level and lower as you become more flexible), opening up in your ankles, knees, and hips. For increased intensity, you can bring your sitting bone to the floor and try to lean back onto your elbows, eventually resting your torso on the floor.

WARM-UP FORWARD BEND

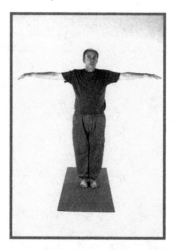

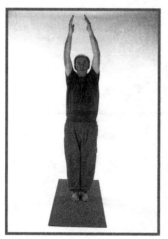
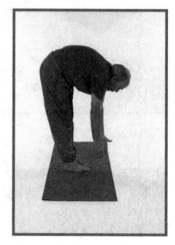

Stand with your feet together in Mountain pose (see page 38). On the inhale, sweep your arms up and over your head. Reach up and then back, stretching through both sides of your torso with your weight in your heels. On the exhale, swan-dive down into a forward bend from the hips, with your arms out to your sides, leading with your chin and chest. Sweep your hands close to the floor and inhale all the way up and back again. Repeat five to six times.

MODIFICATION

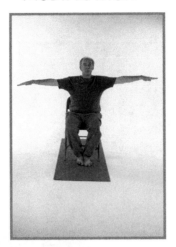

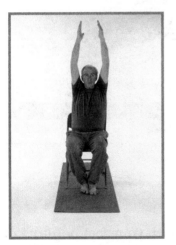
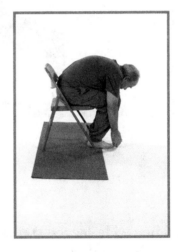

For the chair variation, sit in the chair and face forward with your legs and feet together. Sweep your arms up and then on the exhale, bend down over your legs. On the inhale, come up and reach back. In the beginning, your back may be rounded. As you gain strength, try to come down and up with a straight back.

Note: You should always be aware of any pain or straining in the legs or back and be sure to only do what is comfortable for you

YOGA SQUAT/FORWARD BEND

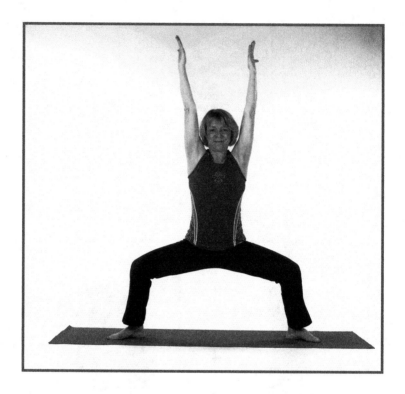

Stand in a wide-legged stance with your feet pointing out. On the inhale, bend your knees and come down halfway while raising your arms into a wide 'V' position.

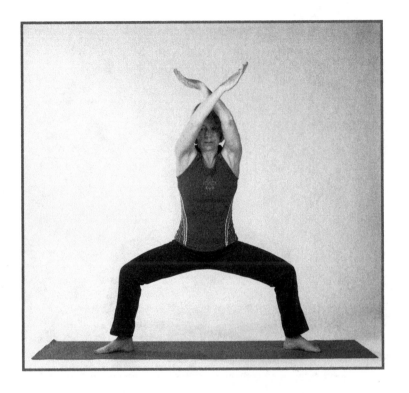

On the exhale, keep your legs where they are and cross your arms above your head.

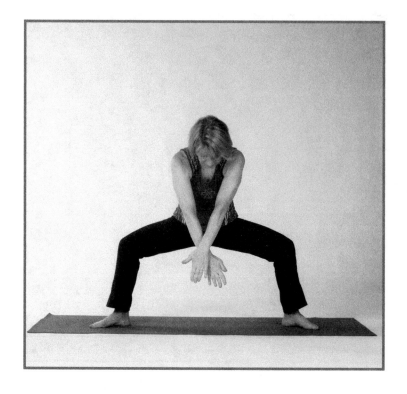

Bend forward halfway, with your arms crossed in front of your body.

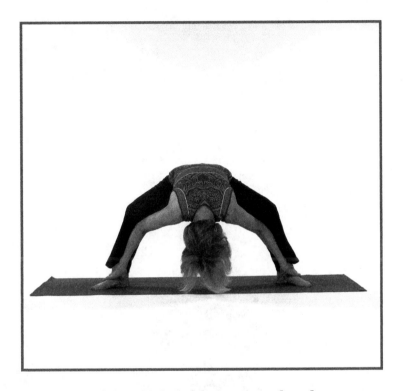

Continue to bend forward and bring your hands to your ankles and your elbows to your knees.

On the next inhale, rise back up into the "V" position. On the exhale, lower down again. Repeat four to five times.

Note: This pose should be done from the hips, not the waist. Once your hands are under your toes, raise your head to keep your spine in alignment and prevent a "hump" in your back.

This pose can also be done with your hands on a chair so that you can straighten your back. As always, use caution and be sure to "listen" to the body—if the pose becomes too difficult, stop or switch to a more gentle variation.

SIDE GATE

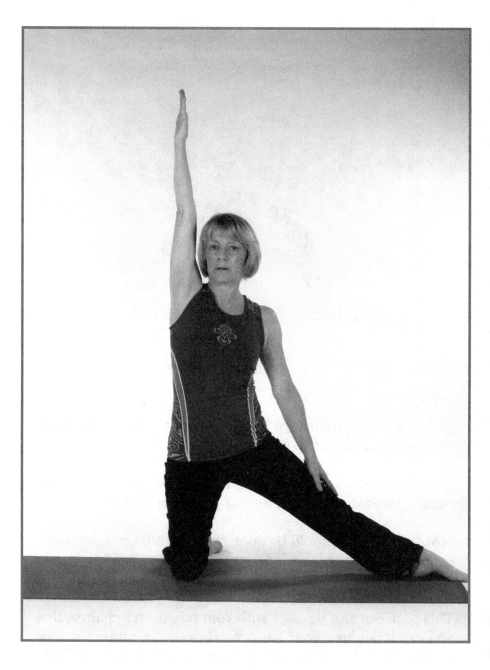

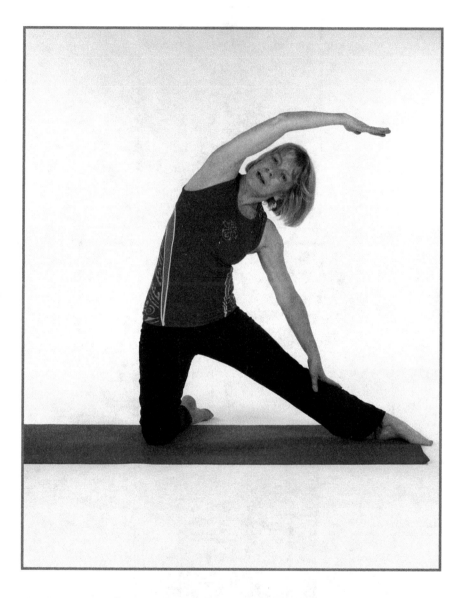

Come to your knees and extend your left leg straight out to the side. On the inhale, raise your right arm straight up. On the exhale, bend to the left, bringing your right arm over your head as your left arm moves down your leg. Hold for five breaths and repeat on the other side.

CHILD

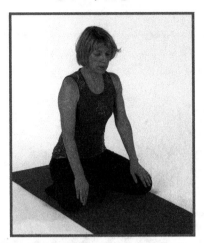

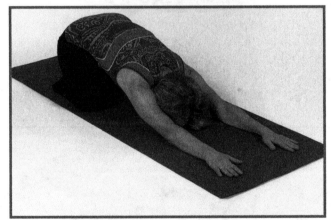

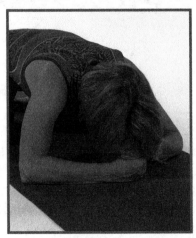

MODIFICATION 1

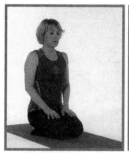 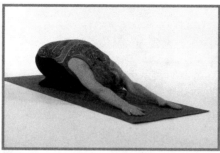 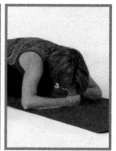

MODIFICATION 2

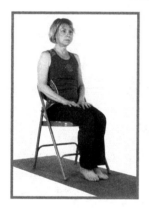 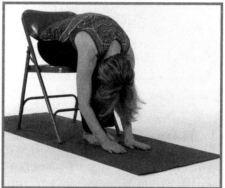

Kneel on the mat, separate your knees, and sit back on your heels (you may also keep your knees together if this is uncomfortable). Bring your body forward, trying to touch your forehead to the floor (if this is difficult, make a fist with your hands and place your forehead on your fists).

For the chair variation, sit with your legs and feet together and roll forward with your arms by your legs and your hands at your feet.

CORPSE

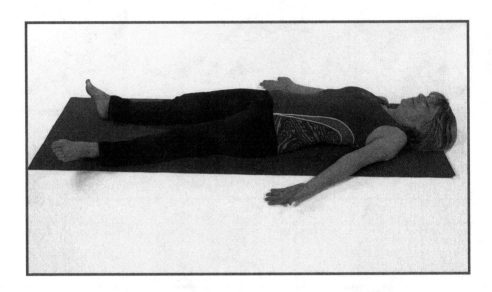

Lie on your back, with your arms extended out from your body and your palms facing up. Keep your legs a little more than hip-width apart to remove any tension from your hips. Close your eyes, bring your chin into the center of your chest, and keep your shoulders relaxed and away from your ears. Breathe deeply into your belly, letting your belly rise and fall with each breath. This pose is recommended at the end of your session to give your body a chance to relax and to allow the previous work from the poses to settle.

CHAPTER 5

GENTLE FLOWS FOR ARTHRITIS

STANDING POSES

POSE	PAGE	EQUIPMENT
Mountain	38	chair (optional)
Hands Under Toes	40	
Warrior I	42	
Warrior II	44	chair (optional)
Warrior III	46	chair (optional)
Triangle	48	block (optional)
Corpse	94	blanket under knees

STANDING BALANCE POSES

POSE	PAGE	EQUIPMENT
Mountain	38	chair (optional)
Tree	52	chair (optional)
Standing Leg Lift	54	chair or strap (optional)
Dancing Shiva	56	chair or strap (optional)
Warrior III	46	chair (optional)
Half Moon	58	block (optional)
Eagle	60	
Corpse	94	blanket under knees

CORE ABDOMINALS

POSE	PAGE	EQUIPMENT
Mountain	38	chair (optional)
Cat and Dog	61	
Downward-Facing Dog	62	wedge under palms
Plank	66	
Upward-Facing Dog	64	
Boat	68	chair (optional)
Locust	70	
Corpse	94	blanket under knees

SHOULDER OPENERS

POSE	PAGE	EQUIPMENT
Mountain	38	chair (optional)
Hands Under Toes	40	
Lateral Stretch	41	block (optional)
Downward-Facing Dog	62	wedge under palms
Triangle	48	block (optional)
Eagle	60	chair (optional)
Sphinx	65	
Bow	74	strap (optional)
Corpse	94	blanket under knees

HIP OPENERS AND TWISTS

POSE	PAGE	EQUIPMENT
Mountain	38	chair (optional)
Half Moon	58	block (optional)
Reverse Triangle	50	block (optional)
Full Squat	76	rolled blanket under heels for support
Seated Twist	78	
Reclined Spinal Twist	80	
Hero	82	block (optional)
Corpse	94	blanket under knees

FORWARD BENDS
AND TWISTS

POSE	PAGE	EQUIPMENT
Mountain	38	chair (optional)
Warm-Up Forward Bend	84	chair (optional)
Yoga Squat/Forward Bend	86	
Seated Twist	78	
Reclined Spinal Twist	80	
Upward-Facing Bent Leg	77	strap (optional)
Side Gate	90	
Corpse	94	blanket under knees

RESTORATIVES

POSE	PAGE	EQUIPMENT
Child	92	chair (optional)
Cat and Dog	61	
Reclined Spinal Twist	80	
Corpse	94	blanket under knees

REFERENCES

American Yoga Association
www.americanyogaassociation.org

Arthritis National Research Foundation
www.curearthritis.org

Arthritis Research Institute of America
www.preventarthritis.org

Mayo Clinic
www.mayoclinic.com

National Institute of Arthritis and Musculoskeletal and Skin Diseases (NIAMS)
www.niams.nih.gov

Rheumatoid Patient Foundation (RPF)
www.rheum4us.org

Yoga Journal
www.yogajournal.com

The Yoga Site
www.yogasite.com

LAURIE SANFORD

Laurie Sanford has practiced yoga for 14 years and is certified under Rob Greenberg, owner of the Yoga for Peace Studio in Margaretville, NY. She has been teaching for eight years and currently provides yoga instruction to adults. Laurie has trained at the Kripalu Center for Yoga and Health, as well as the Himalayan Institute. She currently resides with her husband and daughter in the Catskill Mountains, where they run a weekly newspaper.

NANCY FORSTBAUER

Nancy Forstbauer has been practicing yoga for more than 15 years and has studied under Shiva Rea, leading teacher of Prana Flow Yoga and Yoga Trance Dance. She has also studied with Rodney Yee and his wife Colleen at Kripalu Center for Yoga and Health and with Jill Miller, originator of the *Yoga Tune Up* DVDs. She has also studied Kundalini Yoga with Ana Bret and Ravi Singh, and at Ana Forrest Yoga with Jonathan Bowra. Nancy runs the Stargayzer Yoga studio in Stamford, NY where she holds classes throughout the week. In 2007, she was certified in Yoga Trance Dance. She currently resides in the Catskill Mountains where she works as a Speech Language Pathologist in the area schools.

JO BRIELYN

Jo Brielyn is the co-author of *Combat Fat for Kids: The Complete Plan for Family Fitness, Nutrition, and Health*. Jo is a contributing writer for Hatherleigh Press and has currently completed over 16 nonfiction books about health and wellness. She is a featured author in *Chicken Soup for the Soul: Angels Among Us* and has written numerous articles, short stories and poetry for online and print publications. Jo is the founder, writer and web editor of Creative Kids Ideas and serves as web editor and administrator for GetFitNow.com. In her free time she is also a musician and vocalist with the Christian rock band Common Ground. A western New York native, Jo now resides in Central Florida with her family.